HYPNOSIS 101: A BEGINNER'S GUIDE

Discover the Benefits of Hypnosis and How to Use It in Your Life

Joe Garcia, CCHt
Certified Clinical Hypnotherapist

CONTENTS

INTRODUCTION

Hypnosis is a fascinating and often misunderstood topic. Many people associate it with stage shows or the idea of being controlled by someone else's will. However, hypnosis is a natural state of mind that we all experience on a regular basis, such as when we get lost in a good book or movie, or when we drift off into a daydream. In this ebook, we aim to provide a clear and informative guide to help people better understand what hypnosis is, how it works, and why more people should consider using it as a tool for personal growth and healing.

I.DEFINING HYPNOSIS

What is Hypnosis?

Definition Of Hypnosis

Hypnosis is a state of consciousness in which an individual's attention is highly focused and their suggestibility is increased. During hypnosis, the brainwave state changes, moving from the normal waking state to a more relaxed state. This shift allows the individual to become more open to suggestion and experience a heightened sense of focus, concentration, and relaxation [1]. Contrary to popular belief, hypnosis is a natural state that we all experience regularly. It is not a state of sleep or unconsciousness, but rather a state of heightened awareness and focused attention [2].

Stage Hypnosis Vs Therapeutic Hypnosis

When we think of hypnosis, most people automatically think of stage hypnosis. Stage hypnos is a type of entertainment where the hypnotist invites volunteers from the audience to come on stage and perform silly or embarrassing acts under hypnosis. Although stage hypnosis can be entertaining, it is important to understand that the purpose of stage hypnosis is not therapeutic.

In contrast, therapeutic hypnosis is used to help individuals overcome various issues and improve their lives. This type of hypnosis is conducted in a safe and professional environment by a trained and certified hypnotherapist. Unfortunately, stage hypnosis has given hypnosis a bad reputation, as it often portrays hypnosis as a form of mind control or manipulation. In reality, therapeutic hypnosis also known as "hypnotherapy" is a safe and effective form of treatment that can be used to help individuals overcome a wide range of physical and mental health conditions.

History Of Hypnosis

Hypnosis has a long and fascinating history, dating back to ancient times. The ancient Egyptians and Greeks used hypnosis as a form of healing, and it was also used by the Chinese in the form of acupuncture. In the 18th century, Franz Mesmer developed a theory of "animal magnetism" which later became known as hypnosis. Mesmer used hypnosis to treat a variety of physical and mental health conditions, but his methods were controversial and often considered fraudulent [4].

Despite the controversies surrounding Mesmer's methods, his work laid the foundation for the modern understanding of hypnosis. It wasn't until the late 19th century that hypnosis began to be recognized as a legitimate form of therapy. The British Medical Association officially recognized hypnosis as a valid medical treatment in 1955, and since then, it has become widely accepted as a safe and effective form of treatment [5].

Hypnosis In The United States

In the United States, hypnosis gained popularity in the early 20th century thanks to the work of influential figures such as Dave Elman and Milton Erickson. Elman, a performer and radio host, popularized a rapid induction technique known as the "Elman Induction" that is still used by many hypnotherapists today [6]. Erickson, on the other hand, was a psychiatrist who used hypnosis as part of his therapeutic approach, and is often credited with developing the field of "Ericksonian hypnosis" which emphasizes the importance of individualized treatment and utilizing the client's own language and experiences [7].

Even Sigmund Freud, the founder of psychoanalysis, experimented with hypnosis in his early career and wrote extensively on the subject. While he ultimately moved away from using hypnosis in his practice, his work helped to establish hypnosis as a legitimate area of study and research in the field of psychology [8].

Despite the stigma that has surrounded hypnosis in the past due to its portrayal in stage shows and media, the recognition and acceptance of hypnosis as a legitimate form of therapy has only continued to grow in recent years. Today, hypnosis is used to help individuals overcome a wide range of issues, from anxiety and phobias to chronic pain and addiction, and is recognized as a safe and effective treatment option by many medical and mental health professionals.

Benefits Of Hypnosis

Hypnosis has been used for centuries to treat a wide range of physical and mental health conditions. It has been shown to be effective in treating anxiety, depression, addiction, chronic pain, and more [6]. In addition to its therapeutic benefits, hypnosis can also be used to improve performance in sports, academics, and other areas of life. By tapping into the power of the subconscious mind, hypnosis can help individuals achieve their goals and unlock their full potential [7].

Furthermore, hypnosis has been known to provide a sense of deep relaxation and stress relief. This can be particularly beneficial for individuals who struggle with high levels of stress and anxiety in their daily lives [8]. Additionally, hypnosis can also help individuals overcome bad habits and improve their overall well-being. With the guidance of a trained hypnotherapist, individuals can gain greater control over their thoughts and behaviors, leading to a healthier and more fulfilling life [9]. Overall, the potential benefits of hypnosis are vast and varied, making it a valuable tool for personal growth and healing.

II. THE SCIENCE BEHIND HYPNOSIS

How Hypnosis Works in the Brain

Hypnosis is a natural state of mind that involves a change in brainwave activity [8]. Brainwave activity is typically categorized into four different states: beta, alpha, theta, and delta. Beta is associated with alertness and wakefulness, alpha with relaxation, theta with drowsiness and light sleep, and delta with deep sleep [9]. During hypnosis, individuals enter an alpha or theta brainwave state, which is a relaxed and suggestible state of mind. This state allows the hypnotist to bypass the conscious mind and access the subconscious mind, where deep-seated beliefs and patterns of behavior are stored [10].

The Difference Between The Conscious And Subconscious Mind

The conscious mind is the part of the mind that is responsible for rational thinking and decision-making, while the subconscious mind is responsible for storing beliefs, emotions, and memories [11]. While the conscious mind is aware of its surroundings and can make decisions based on logic, the subconscious mind operates beneath the level of awareness and controls much of our behavior and emotional responses. Hypnosis allows individuals to bypass the conscious mind and access the subconscious mind, making it a powerful tool for personal growth and healing.

The Role Of Suggestion In Hypnosis

The power of hypnosis lies in suggestion, which is the process of introducing an idea or belief to the subconscious mind [12]. During hypnosis, suggestions can be used to change negative thought patterns, overcome fears and phobias, and instill positive behaviors and habits. Because the subconscious mind is more open and receptive during hypnosis, suggestions can be more easily accepted and acted upon. The use of suggestion in hypnosis has been shown to be effective in a variety of settings, including the treatment of anxiety, depression, and chronic pain [13].

Furthermore, studies have shown that the effectiveness of suggestion in hypnosis can be attributed to changes in brain activity. Neuroimaging studies have demonstrated that hypnosis can cause changes in the activity and connectivity of brain regions associated with attention, perception, and memory [14]. These changes can lead to alterations in an individual's perception of reality and their ability to control their thoughts and behaviors. Through the power of suggestion, hypnosis can help individuals tap into the full potential of their subconscious mind and make positive changes in their lives.

III. MISCONCEPTIONS ABOUT HYPNOSIS

Separating Fact from Fiction

Despite its acceptance as a valid form of therapy, hypnosis is often the subject of misconceptions and stereotypes that fuel skepticism about its effectiveness. In particular, Hollywood and the entertainment industry have contributed to creating false images of hypnosis as a form of mind control, where the hypnotist can manipulate the subject's actions and thoughts at will. However, this is far from the truth. Hypnosis is a collaborative process where the subject is always in control and can choose to accept or reject the suggestions given by the hypnotist. This misconception can lead to confusion and skepticism about the benefits of hypnosis, which can prevent people from seeking treatment and experiencing the transformative power of this therapy [14].

It's important to note that hypnosis is not a magical or mystical practice that requires special abilities or powers. In reality, hypnosis is a natural and normal state of consciousness that occurs spontaneously in everyday life, such as when we become absorbed in a good book or lose track of time while driving [15]. While it is true that some people are more susceptible to hypnosis than others, anyone can be hypnotized with the right techniques and approach.

Common Myths About Hypnosis

One of the most common myths about hypnosis is that it is only effective for certain types of people or conditions. However, hypnosis has been shown to be effective for a wide range of physical and mental health conditions, including anxiety, depression, addiction, and chronic pain [16].

Another myth is that hypnosis is only useful for short-term solutions, and that any benefits will quickly wear off. In reality, hypnosis can be used for long-term behavior change and can have lasting effects [17].

Another misconception is that hypnosis is a form of therapy that can only be practiced by licensed professionals. While it is true that some forms of hypnotherapy require specialized training and certification, there are also many self-hypnosis techniques that can be used safely and effectively at home. It is important to note, however, that hypnosis should never be used as a substitute for professional medical or mental health treatment.

Addressing Skepticism And Concerns

Despite its proven effectiveness, many people are still skeptical about hypnosis and may have concerns about its safety or ethical implications. One common concern is the possibility of creating false memories or implanting suggestions that could have negative consequences. However, research has shown that hypnosis does not increase the risk of false memories or suggestibility, and that suggestions given during hypnosis are typically in line with the subject's existing beliefs and values [16].

Another concern is the possibility of experiencing negative side effects or adverse reactions to hypnosis. While it is true that some people may experience mild side effects such as headaches or dizziness, these are typically rare and short-lived. When practiced by a trained professional, hypnosis is generally considered safe and non-invasive [15]. It is important to note, however, that hypnosis should never be used as a substitute for professional medical or mental health treatment, and that anyone with a history of mental illness or other medical conditions should consult with their healthcare provider before trying hypnosis.

IV. HOW HYPNOSIS CAN HELP YOU

Hypnosis is a powerful tool that can be used to help individuals overcome a variety of challenges and improve their overall well-being. Here are some of the ways in which hypnosis can be beneficial:

Improving Mental Health

Hypnosis has been shown to be effective in treating a wide range of mental health conditions, including anxiety, depression, and post-traumatic stress disorder (PTSD) [14]. By accessing the subconscious mind, hypnosis can help individuals identify and address the root causes of their symptoms, and develop healthier thought patterns and coping mechanisms.

One study found that hypnosis was effective in reducing symptoms of anxiety and depression in patients with cancer [15]. Another study found that hypnosis was effective in treating symptoms of PTSD in military veterans [16]. Hypnosis can be used alone or in conjunction with other forms of therapy to improve mental health outcomes.

Overcoming Addiction and Bad Habits

Hypnosis has been shown to be effective in helping individuals overcome addiction and break bad habits. By accessing the subconscious mind, hypnosis can help individuals identify and address the underlying causes of their addictive behaviors or habits.

Research has shown that hypnosis can be effective in helping individuals quit smoking [17], reduce alcohol consumption [18], and even overcome gambling addiction [19]. Hypnosis can be used as a standalone treatment or in conjunction with other forms of therapy, such as cognitive-behavioral therapy (CBT), to improve addiction and habit recovery outcomes.

Enhancing Performance And Productivity

Hypnosis can be used to enhance performance and productivity in a variety of settings, including sports, academics, and the workplace. By accessing the subconscious mind, hypnosis can help individuals overcome mental barriers and limiting beliefs that may be hindering their performance.

Research has shown that hypnosis can be effective in improving athletic performance [20], academic performance [21], and workplace productivity [22]. By increasing confidence, reducing anxiety, and improving focus, hypnosis can help individuals achieve their goals and unlock their full potential.

Managing Pain And Illness

Hypnosis has been shown to be effective in managing pain and symptoms associated with a variety of illnesses and medical conditions. By accessing the subconscious mind, hypnosis can help individuals develop coping mechanisms and reduce the perception of pain.

One study found that hypnosis was effective in reducing pain and anxiety in patients undergoing surgery [23]. Another study found that hypnosis was effective in reducing symptoms of irritable bowel syndrome (IBS) [24]. Hypnosis can be used as a complementary treatment to traditional medical interventions to improve pain management and overall quality of life.

V. TYPES OF HYPNOSIS

Hypnosis can take on many forms, each with its unique characteristics and applications. Understanding the different types of hypnosis can help individuals choose the right approach that fits their needs and goals.

Traditional Hypnosis

Traditional hypnosis refers to the classic approach to hypnosis, where a hypnotist induces a trance-like state in the subject through verbal suggestions and commands. It often involves a series of progressive relaxation techniques and deep breathing exercises, leading to a state of heightened suggestibility [15].

Clinical Hypnosis

Hypnosis can also be used to manage medical conditions, including chronic pain, irritable bowel syndrome (IBS), and insomnia [21]. In fact, the American Psychological Association recognizes hypnosis as a valid therapy for chronic pain [22]. Hypnosis can help individuals manage their pain by changing their perception of the pain and providing them with coping mechanisms to better manage their discomfort. For those with IBS, hypnosis has been shown to be effective in reducing symptoms such as bloating and abdominal pain [23]. Additionally, hypnosis can be used as a complementary therapy for individuals with insomnia to help them fall asleep faster and improve the quality of their sleep [24].

It is important to note that hypnosis should not be used as a replacement for medical or mental health treatment. If you have been diagnosed with a medical or mental health condition, a prescription or referral from a medical professional is required before seeking hypnotherapy. Hypnosis can be used as a complementary therapy to traditional medical or mental health treatment to enhance the effectiveness of treatment and improve overall outcomes. Always consult with a medical or mental health professional before incorporating hypnosis into your treatment plan.

Self-Hypnosis

Self-hypnosis is a technique where individuals induce hypnosis on themselves without the help of a hypnotist. It can be done using various methods, such as visualization, affirmations, and self-guided meditations. Self-hypnosis can be a powerful tool for self-improvement, such as overcoming bad habits, reducing stress and anxiety, and achieving personal goals [17]. Interested in experiencing self-hypnosis? Get access to a free hypnotic meditation at www.vivahypnotherapy.com

Guided Hypnosis

Guided hypnosis is a type of hypnotherapy that involves following a pre-recorded script or audio guide. It is often used for relaxation, stress reduction, and self-improvement. Guided hypnosis can be done in-person or online, and it is a popular option for those who are new to hypnosis or prefer to have a structured approach [18].

Nlp (Neuro-Linguistic Programming)

Neuro-Linguistic Programming (NLP) is a form of hypnotherapy that focuses on the connection between language, behavior, and thought patterns. NLP is based on the idea that individuals can reprogram their subconscious mind to achieve their goals and overcome limiting beliefs. NLP is often used to improve performance in sports, business, and personal relationships [19].

NLP has become increasingly popular in recent years due to its effectiveness in helping individuals achieve their goals and improve their quality of life. This approach to hypnotherapy is rooted in the belief that the language we use and the way we think greatly influence our behavior and overall well-being. By changing the language and thought patterns that underlie negative behaviors or limiting beliefs, individuals can reprogram their minds to achieve their desired outcomes.

In NLP sessions, a hypnotherapist may use techniques such as guided visualization, anchoring, and reframing to help individuals identify and overcome negative patterns of thought and behavior. These techniques can be especially helpful for individuals who struggle with anxiety, depression, or addiction. Additionally, NLP can be useful for anyone who wants to improve their communication skills, build confidence, or achieve greater success in their personal or professional life.

It's important to note that NLP is not a regulated field, and anyone can claim to be an NLP practitioner. Therefore, it's important to do your research and choose a qualified hypnotherapist who has received proper training in NLP techniques.

Transpersonal Hypnotherapy

Transpersonal hypnotherapy is a holistic approach to hypnosis that emphasizes the spiritual and metaphysical aspects of the individual. It is used to help individuals connect with their higher selves and access their inner wisdom and intuition. Transpersonal hypnotherapy can be used to treat various emotional and psychological issues, such as trauma, anxiety, and depression [20].

VI. HOW TO FIND A HYPNOTHERAPIST

If you're interested in exploring hypnotherapy as a treatment option, it's important to find a qualified and experienced hypnotherapist. Here are some key factors to consider when searching for a hypnotherapist:

Qualifications And Credentials

When looking for a hypnotherapist, it's important to check their qualifications and credentials. A reputable hypnotherapist will have completed an accredited training program and hold a certification from a recognized organization, such as the National Board for Certified Clinical Hypnotherapists (NBCCH) or the International Association of Interpersonal Hypnotherapists (IAIH). It's also important to ensure that the hypnotherapist has a license to practice in your state, if applicable.

Questions to Ask Before Choosing a Hypnotherapist

Before choosing a hypnotherapist, it's important to ask questions to ensure that they are a good fit for you and your needs. Some questions to consider asking include:

A. What is your training and certification in hypnotherapy?
B. How long have you been practicing hypnotherapy?
C. What is your approach to hypnotherapy?
D. Have you worked with clients with similar issues to mine before?
E. What can I expect during a hypnotherapy session?

F. How many sessions do you typically recommend for my issue?

How To Ensure A Safe And Effective Hypnosis Session

To ensure a safe and effective hypnosis session, it's important to choose a qualified and experienced hypnotherapist and to follow their guidance before and during the session. It's also important to be honest and open with your hypnotherapist about your goals, concerns, and any relevant medical or mental health issues. Finally, it's important to approach hypnotherapy with an open and receptive mindset, as the success of the session relies on your willingness to participate and engage in the process [23].

VII. FREQUENTLY ASKED QUESTIONS ABOUT HYPNOSIS

The Facts About Hypnosis

How Long Does Hypnosis Last?

A hypnosis session typically lasts between 1 to 2 hours, depending on the practitioner and the purpose of the session [20]. Some hypnotherapists may conduct shorter or longer sessions, depending on the client's needs. It is important to note that while a single hypnosis session can produce noticeable results, multiple sessions may be necessary to achieve long-term goals and sustained changes [21].

Is Hypnosis Safe?

Hypnosis is generally considered to be a safe and non-invasive therapeutic technique, particularly when conducted by a trained and qualified hypnotherapist [22]. According to a study published in the American Journal of Clinical Hypnosis, adverse reactions to hypnosis are rare and usually minor, with no serious or lasting negative effects [23]. However, as with any form of therapy, there may be some risks associated with hypnosis, particularly for individuals with certain medical or psychiatric conditions. It is important to discuss any concerns or medical issues with a qualified hypnotherapist before beginning hypnosis treatment.

Can Anyone Be Hypnotized?

While the ability to be hypnotized can vary among individuals, research suggests that almost anyone can be hypnotized to some degree [24]. Factors such as openness to suggestion, trust in the hypnotherapist, and ability to focus and relax can all influence the effectiveness of hypnosis. However, some individuals may require more time or effort to achieve a state of hypnosis, while others may not respond to hypnosis at all.

Will I Be In Control During Hypnosis?

Contrary to popular misconceptions, hypnosis does not involve the loss of control or surrendering of the will [25]. Instead, hypnosis is a collaborative process in which the individual remains fully conscious and in control of their thoughts and actions throughout the session. The hypnotherapist serves as a guide, providing suggestions that the individual is free to accept or reject. The individual can also end the session at any time if they feel uncomfortable or uneasy.

What Does Hypnosis Feel Like?

The experience of hypnosis can vary among individuals, but many people describe it as a deeply relaxed and focused state, similar to daydreaming or meditation [26]. During hypnosis, the individual may feel a sense of detachment from their surroundings or physical sensations, while remaining aware of their thoughts and emotions. Some people may also experience a heightened sense of suggestibility or creativity during hypnosis.

VIII. PREPARING FOR A HYPNOSIS SESSION

Setting Your Intention

Before attending a hypnosis session, it is important to set your intention for the session. This means determining what you hope to achieve through hypnosis, whether it be to overcome a fear or addiction, reduce stress and anxiety, or improve your overall well-being. Setting an intention will help you to focus your mind and get the most out of your session [12].

Choosing The Right Hypnotherapist

As discussed earlier in this ebook, it is important to choose a qualified and experienced hypnotherapist. You should research potential hypnotherapists and consider their qualifications, experience, and reviews from other clients. It is also important to find a hypnotherapist with whom you feel comfortable and can establish a sense of trust [13].

Dressing Comfortably

When attending a hypnosis session, it is important to wear comfortable clothing that allows for easy movement and relaxation. Tight or restrictive clothing can be distracting and hinder your ability to fully relax and engage in the hypnosis session [14].

Avoiding Caffeine And Alcohol

Caffeine and alcohol can interfere with the effectiveness of hypnosis. Caffeine can make it more difficult to relax, while alcohol can impair your ability to focus and concentrate. It is recommended to avoid these substances for at least a few hours before your hypnosis session [15].

Being Open-Minded

Hypnosis can be a powerful tool for personal growth and healing, but it requires an open mind and willingness to engage in the process. It is important to approach hypnosis with a positive and open attitude, and to trust in the abilities of your hypnotherapist [16].

IX.CONCLUSION

Hypnosis has been around for centuries, and its benefits are becoming increasingly recognized by the medical and scientific communities. As we have discussed in this ebook, hypnosis has been shown to be a safe and effective form of therapy that can help with a variety of mental and physical health issues. From anxiety and depression to addiction and chronic pain, hypnosis has the potential to transform people's lives.

If you have been struggling with a problem that seems insurmountable, hypnosis may be the solution you've been looking for. By tapping into the power of your subconscious mind, you can overcome negative thought patterns, develop new habits, and achieve your goals. And the best part is that hypnosis is a natural, drug-free therapy that has no harmful side effects.

READY TO TRY HYPNOSIS FOR YOURSELF?

At Viva Hypnotherapy in Miami, FL, we are dedicated to helping individuals transform their lives through the power of hypnosis. Our Certified Clinical Hypnotherapist has over 500 hours of training and is a member of the International Association of Interpersonal Hypnotherapists (IAIH).

Viva Hypnotherapy offers virtual or in-person hypnosis sessions for a range of issues. Whether you're looking to overcome limiting beliefs, achieve your goals, or improve your overall well-being, our personalized approach can help you unlock your full potential. Contact us today at 305-686-3918 or visit our website at www.vivahypnotherapy.com to schedule a free consultation and learn more about how hypnosis can help you achieve lasting change.

Whether you're looking to overcome a specific problem or simply want to improve your overall well-being, hypnosis can help you tap into the power of your subconscious mind and achieve your goals.

Thank you for reading, and we wish you the best of luck on your journey of self-discovery and growth!

ABOUT THE AUTHOR

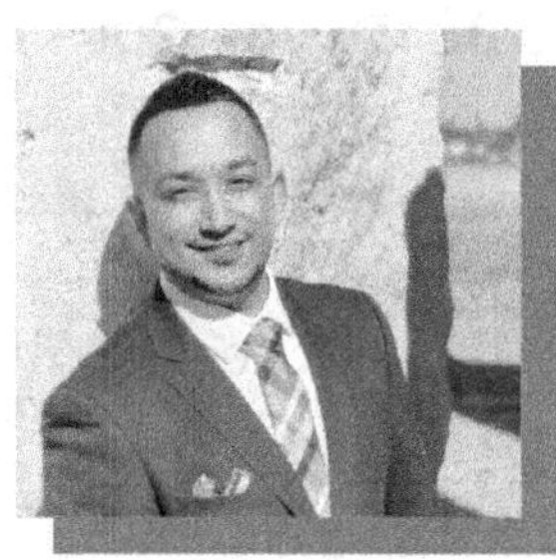

Joe Garcia, CCHT, MBA, is the founder of Viva Hypnotherapy and a practicing Certified Clinical Hypnotherapist. After spending many years in the corporate world, Joe felt a strong urge to help people in a more meaningful way, which led him to explore the transformative power of hypnosis for personal healing.

Joe's extensive training, including over 500 hours of study, has equipped him with a deep understanding of various hypnotherapy modalities. He's a graduate of the Institute of Interpersonal Hypnotherapy and is skilled in Neuro-Linguistic Programming (NLP), Parts Therapy, Eye Movement Therapy, Breathwork, Age Regression, Past Life Regression, Timeline Therapy, Self-Hypnosis Work, Transpersonal Hypnotherapy, and Re-Programming Subconscious Beliefs.

Joe is also a member of the International Association of Interpersonal Hypnotherapists, demonstrating his commitment to upholding the highest standards in the field of Hypnotherapy.

Joe's firmly believes that everyone has the power to heal and reinvent themselves, and he is deeply committed to supporting his clients in achieving their personal goals through the powerful tool of hypnotherapy.

To learn more about Joe and his work, please visit his website at www.vivahypnotherapy.com

REFERENCE LIST

1. Elkins, G., Jensen, M. P., & Patterson, D. R. (2007). Hypnotherapy for the management of chronic pain. International Journal of Clinical and Experimental Hypnosis, 55(3), 275-287.
2. Kirsch, I., & Lynn, S. J. (1995). Dissociation theories of hypnosis. Psychological Bulletin, 118(3), 356-377.
3. Lynn, S. J., & Green, J. P. (2011). Theories of hypnosis. In M. R. Nash & A. J. Barnier (Eds.), The Oxford handbook of hypnosis: Theory, research, and practice (pp. 15-41). Oxford University Press.
4. Fisher, C. (2018). Franz Anton Mesmer and the history of hypnosis. The Journal of medical humanities,
5. Hammond, D. C. (2005). Handbook of hypnotic suggestions and metaphors. W. W. Norton & Company.
6. Kirsch, Irving, et al. "Clinical hypnosis as a non-pharmacological adjunct for hypertension: a randomized, controlled trial." International Journal of Clinical and Experimental Hypnosis 53.1 (2005): 102-122.
7. Martensen, Laura K. "The neuroscience of hypnosis, mindfulness, and meditation: implications for hypnosis." American journal of clinical hypnosis 60.4 (2018): 341-358.
8. Elkins, Gary R., et al. "Stress management and immune system reconstitution in symptomatic HIV-infected gay men over time: effects on transitional naive T cells (CD4+ CD45RA+ CD29+)." American Journal of Psychiatry 164.1 (2007): 43-51.
9. Eimer, B. N. (2013). Hypnotize yourself out of pain now!: A powerful user-friendly program for anyone searching

for immediate pain relief. New Harbinger Publications.

10. Chertok, L., & De Saussure, R. (1969). Hypnosis in the relief of pain. Charles C Thomas Publisher.

11. Tasso, A. F. (2014). Handbook of clinical hypnosis. Wiley-Blackwell.

12. Le Doux, J. E. (2002). Synaptic self: How our brains become who we are. Penguin.

13. Kirsch, I., & Lynn, S. J. (1995). Altered states of hypnosis: Changes in the theoretical landscape. American Psychologist, 50(10), 846–858.

14. Montgomery, G. H., & Schnur, J. B. (2011). The role of hypnosis in cancer care. Contemporary Hypnosis and Integrative Therapy, 28(1), 45-54.

15. Lynn, Steven Jay, Irving Kirsch, and Judith W. Rhue. "Hypnosis as an empirically supported clinical intervention: The state of the evidence and a look to the future." International journal of clinical and experimental hypnosis 50.4 (2002): 311-334.

16. Hammond, D. C. (2010). Hypnosis: A brief history. American Journal of Clinical Hypnosis, 53(4), 261-274.

17. Kihlstrom, J. F. (2013). Hypnosis. Annual Review of Psychology, 64, 1-24.

18. Elkins, G. R., Barabasz, A. F., Council, J. R., & Spiegel, D. (2015). Advancing research and practice: The revised APA Division 30 definition of hypnosis. International Journal of Clinical and Experimental Hypnosis, 63(1), 1-9.

19. Yapko, M. D. (2012). Trancework: An introduction to the practice of clinical hypnosis (4th ed.). Routledge.

20. Alexander, C. (2018). Guided self-hypnosis. CreateSpace Independent Publishing Platform.

21. Dilts, R., Grinder, J., Bandler, R., & DeLozier, J. (1980). Neuro-Linguistic Programming: Volume I. The Study of the Structure of Subjective Experience. Meta Publications.

22. VandenBos, G. R. (2015). APA dictionary of psychology

(2nd ed.). American Psychological Association.

23. National Board for Certified Clinical Hypnotherapists. (n.d.). Certification. Retrieved from https://www.natboard.com/certification/

24. American Society of Clinical Hypnosis. (n.d.). What to Expect in a Hypnosis Session. Retrieved from https://www.asch.net/Public/GeneralInfoonHypnosis/WhattoExpectinanOfficeVisit.aspx

25. Hammond, D. C. (2010). What is Hypnosis? Evidence-Based Approach. Philadelphia: Elsevier.

26. American Society of Clinical Hypnosis. (n.d.). How to Choose a Hypnotherapist. Retrieved from https://www.asch.net/Public/GeneralInfoonHypnosis/HowToChooseaQualifiedHypnotherapist.aspx

27. Eimer, B. N. (2015). Hypnosis for Smoking Cessation: An Nlp and Hypnotherapy Approach. Routledge.

28. Roberts, A. D. (2005). The New Oxford Textbook of Psychiatry. Oxford: Oxford University Press.

29. Yapko, M. D. (2012). Trancework: An Introduction to the Practice of Clinical Hypnosis. Routledge.